Healthy Lifestyle Against Diabetes

1st. Edition

Control, prevent and reverse your diabetes. A nutritional and mindset approach

Amie Armstrong

medical or professional advice. The content of this book has been derived from various sources. Please consult a licensed professional before attempting any techniques outlined in this book.

By reading this document, the reader agrees that under no circumstances is the author responsible for any losses, direct or indirect, which are incurred as a result of the use of information contained within this document, including, but not limited to, —errors, omissions, or inaccuracies.

Dedicatory

Dedicated to the people that are fighting against the

diabetes

TABLE OF CONTENTS

INTRODUCTION

Understanding the basic concepts of diabetes is the first step that must be taken to have control of your health. Let's see what causes diabetes, some of the most common symptoms, the benefits of living a healthy life, and what to do if you are newly diagnosed with diabetes.

Diabetes is a disease that occurs when the level of glucose in the blood, also known as blood sugar, is too high. Blood glucose is the main source of energy and comes from food. Insulin, a hormone produced by the pancreas, helps the glucose in food enter the cells to be used as energy. Sometimes the body does not produce enough or does not produce any insulin or does not use it properly and the glucose stays in the blood and does not reach the cells.

Over time, too much glucose in the blood can cause health problems . Although diabetes has no cure, the person with diabetes can take steps to control their disease and stay healthy.

Sometimes people who have diabetes say they have "a little high sugar" or have "prediabetes." These terms make us think that the person does not really have diabetes or that their case is less serious. However, all cases of diabetes are serious.

Diabetes mellitus is a metabolic disease characterized by elevated blood sugar (glucose) levels.

The glucose that circulates in the blood is called glycemia .

The increase in blood glucose is the result of defects in insulin secretion , in its action or both. The insulin is a hormone made by the pancreas and which allows cells to utilize the glucose in the blood as an energy source.

Insulin production, insulin action, or both, causes an increase in blood glucose levels (hyperglycemia). If not adequately controlled, in the long term, the continuous presence of high glucose in the blood can cause alterations in the function of various organs, especially the eyes, kidneys, nerves, heart and blood vessels.

CHAPTER 1

The Different Types Of Diabetes

In 1998, 143 million people around the world were diabetic. And if we believe the forecasts, there will be 300 million patients in 2025. Diabetes is a disease that, without appropriate treatment, can cause serious complications. Characterized by a permanent excess of sugar in the blood, diabetes can be of different types: type 1 and type 2. What is the difference? What role does insulin play for everyone? Answers from experts.

Diabetes is a chronic disease that persists throughout life. The correct management of the disease by the patient himself, with the help of his doctor, must avoid the complications. Diabetes is responsible for poor health conditions and premature death.

Diabetes type 1 and type 2 diabetes: what are the differences?

TYPE 1	TYPE 2
- Type 1, insulin-dependent diabetes (IDDM) also known as "lean" diabetes because one of the first symptoms is weight loss, or "juvenile" because it affects young people.	- Type 2, non-insulin-dependent diabetes mellitus (NIDDM), also known as "fat" diabetes or diabetes mellitus, since it often occurs in middle age in overweight people.
- It accounts for about 10% of cases and is treated compulsorily by insulin.	- It accounts for about 90% of cases and is treated by diet, plus drugs taken orally if necessary, and possibly insulin, after a few years of evolution.

Why this imbalance in sugar during diabetes?

Diabetes is a disorder of assimilation, use and storage of sugars brought by food. During digestion, the food we eat is transformed into sugar, which is essential for the cells of the body to function. It is insulin , a hormone produced by the pancreas , that regulates the amount of sugar stored or "burned" in cells. After crossing the intestinal wall, the sugar is found in the bloodstream, increasing blood sugar. This signal is detected by particular cells of the pancreas (beta cells of islets of Langerhans), which then secrete insulin. The presence of insulin in the blood is itself perceived by the cells of the liver, muscles and fatty tissues, which in response begin to consume glucose or store it for later use. Hence a return to normal blood sugar level.

Insulin: its role in glucose uptake by the cell

In The Person Without Diabetes

1 - Released by the pancreas, insulin allows the absorption of glucose by the cells. To do this, it binds to a specific receptor of the cell that activates a surface protein whose role is the transport of glucose inwards.

2 - Via this activated transporter, the glucose enters the cell where it is converted into energy.

3 - The blood glucose level (glycemia) remains stable.

In The Diabetic Person

1 - Insulin is produced in insufficient quantity (type 1 diabetes) or can not bind to its receptor (type 2 diabetes) leaving the carrier inactive

2 - Glucose does not enter the cell and remains in the bloodstream . The glucose level is not regulated.

Diabetes is caused by insufficient secretion and / or action of insulin. That pancreatic cells are destroyed (insulin-dependent diabetes in young patients) or exhausted by too rich diet and genetic predisposition (diabetes mellitus adult subject), and the lack of insulin prevents the proper passage of sugar from the blood to the tissue. The blood sugar then remains high after meals.

Diagnosis of diabetes

Normal blood glucose is less than 1.10g / l on an empty stomach and less than 1.40g / l after a meal. Diabetes is defined as fasting blood glucose greater than 1.26 g / l twice. Glycosuria is the presence of glucose in the urine. It appears when the blood glucose is above 60g / l. Between these two cases, there is an intermediate situation to indicate a strong predisposition to become diabetic.

CHAPTER 2

How To Control Your Diabetes

For many, the diagnosis of diabetes should be made as soon as possible. In general, there are two pillars of diabetes control: regular checking of blood sugar levels (known as blood sugar) and healthy, active living. Drug treatments, which usually consist of injecting insulin, also help maintain normal blood glucose levels and manage the manifestations of diabetes. Follow our tips to effectively control your diabetes and live a healthy and happy life. However, keep in mind that these tips are only for informational purposes and do not replace the advice of specialists.

Plan the treatment of your diabetes

Type 1 diabetes

Whatever the situation, consult your doctor first. Type 1 diabetes, also known as juvenile diabetes, is a chronic disease that, contrary to what its name indicates, can occur at any age. This form of diabetes usually appears abruptly, with no warning signs. If left untreated, it can become dangerous and even fatal. Therefore, it is extremely important to consult and be followed by a doctor who will provide you with advice and assistance during your treatment.

Neither type 1 diabetes nor type 2 diabetes can be fully cured. Nevertheless, by following a long-term treatment, or even for life, you can effectively control your illness and live a normal life. Your treatment will be all the more effective if you start it early. If you think you have diabetes, see a doctor as soon as possible. Because manifestations of type 1 diabetes can be serious, a short hospitalization following the diagnosis is ☐uite common.

Take your insulin dose every day.

The body of people with type 1 diabetes is unable to produce insulin. This protein has a hypoglycemic effect, that is to say, it regulates down the blood sugar level. Without insulin injection, the condition of the patient with juvenile diabetes will worsen until death. For this reason, type 1 diabetes is also known as insulin-dependent diabetes mellitus (IDDM). The amount of insulin to be taken is prescribed according to the patient, taking into account various parameters such as its size, its diet, its level of activity but also genetic factors. It is therefore important to consult a doctor, who will do all the necessary tests to define the appropriate treatment. Insulin is available in many forms, each specifically formulated to meet a specific need.

Fast insulin (to be taken at mealtimes). This fast-acting insulin should be taken before meals to prevent an increase in blood glucose following the meal.

Basal insulin. This insulin is used as a background treatment. Administered once or twice a day, it helps keep blood glucose levels off meal periods.

Premixed insulin. It is a combination of fast insulin and basal insulin. It can be taken before breakfast and dinner. It keeps your blood sugar under control all day and at mealtimes.

Exercise.

The regular practice of a sport has many beneficial effects: weight loss, increased strength, endurance and energy, well-defined silhouette, good mood ... But playing sports is even more important for people with diabetes. Indeed, the regular practice of a sport has a hypoglycemic effect, which can last up to 24 hours. As the danger of diabetes resides precisely in increasing blood sugar levels, it is important for diabetics to maintain their physical condition.

It is recommended to exercise several times a week. The ideal is to combine cardio, strength training, stretching and maintaining balance.

Nevertheless, it must be ensured that your blood sugar level is not too low either. Indeed, below a certain level, the body is in a state of hypoglycemia and is no longer able to produce the energy necessary for vital functions and muscle maintenance. The patient may then experience severe fatigue, dizziness and even fainting. To guard against the risk of hypoglycemia, always have a sweet product or a high-carb drink (such as a soda or energy drink) on you.

Reduce the sources of stress.

Whether stress is mental or physical, it is recognized that it can cause fluctuations in blood sugar levels. Continuous and prolonged stress can increase your blood sugar in the long run, forcing you to take a heavier treatment and exercise more.

Do not let stress settle: avoid potentially stressful situations as much as possible, get enough sleep, exercise and do not hesitate to talk to your friends about your problems.

Other solutions exist to help you manage your stress. Indeed, you can follow a therapy or do some meditation. Know also that caffeine is a stressful substance, so you must banish it from your diet. Finally, some hobbies can be beneficial.

At menstruation or menopause, change your treatment.

Diabetic women face an additional problem related to their menstrual cycle. Most women report that their blood glucose levels increase during the premenstrual period, which re□uires compensation for more fre□uent insulin injections and more intense exercise. However, the change in blood glucose levels during the menstrual cycle differ from one woman to another, so ask your doctor or gynecologist for advice.

It is also necessary to be vigilant at the age of menopause. Indeed, at this time, the control of blood glucose by the body can change. As a result, many women report that, at menopause, their blood sugar levels are difficult to control because they are unpredictable. This problem is compounded by a series of side effects experienced by postmenopausal women (weight gain, loss of sleep, vaginal problems ...), a source of stress and therefore an increase in blood sugar. Anticipate these disturbances as much as possible by planning a specific treatment with your doctor as soon as menopausal symptoms are felt.

Type 2 diabetes

Consult your doctor before starting your treatment.

The body of patients with type 2 diabetes is capable of producing insulin, which explains that it is also called non-insulin-dependent (NIDDM). However, depending on the case, either the amount of protein produced is insufficient or the protein is not functional. In fact, type 2 diabetes is triggered gradually and its symptoms make it less dangerous than type 1 diabetes. In some cases, it is asymptomatic, ie the patient does not feel it. not and therefore does not necessarily know that he has it. This explains that the treatment is also, unless exception, less heavy. However, as with type 1 diabetes, it is essential to consult your doctor before starting any treatment.

If possible, control your blood sugar using a proper diet and exercise.

As already mentioned, type 2 diabetics produce insulin, which allows them to live with their diabetes without the injection of artificial insulin. In general, patients can manage their illness by following an adapted food and sports program. They have to reduce their sugar intake, maintain their weight and play sports regularly. In some cases, the patient may even lead a normal life without following a specific diet or exercising particularly.

However, some cases of type 2 diabetes require special attention and even additional insulin or drug treatment.

Note: Refer to the sections below for more information on diets and drug treatments.

Prepare for your treatment to change over time.

Type 2 diabetes is a progressive disease that usually gets worse over time. According to studies conducted on the subject, this is due to a gradual but rapid wear of Langerhans cells (insulin producers) who are increasingly solicited because of their low production of the protein. As a result, patients with type 2 diabetes may begin with simple treatment that will become more and more cumbersome. The aggravation of the disease is sometimes independent of the patient's life choices.

Although type 2 diabetes is more manageable than type 1 diabetes, you should still keep in touch with your doctor for regular checkups and anticipate any progression of the disease.

In case of morbid obesity, you can resort to bariatric surgery. Obesity is an aggravating factor of diabetes in general. But it is one of the most important causes of type 2 diabetes (which explains its name of fatty diabetes). The added stress of obesity makes controlling the disease even more complicated. When the patient, type 2 diabetic, is also morbidly obese (Body Mass Index greater than 35), the doctor will direct him to obesity surgery (or bariatric surgery), intended to rapidly reduce body mass. . This specific surgery comes in two main techniques:

Gastric Bypass: This involves keeping only a small gastric pouch (no larger than one inch) and reducing the size of the bowel. By reducing the size of the digestive system and its ability to absorb nutrients, this technique allows the patient to lose weight dramatically and permanently.

Gastric banding (or gastroplasty): A ring is placed to enclose the top of the stomach, which reduces its ability to store food. This operation is reversible (the ring can be removed) and adjustable (the size of the ring and its position can be modified).

CHAPTER 3

How To Prevent And Treat Diabetes With Natural Medicine

Insulin is a hormone produced by the body that is used to control the level of sugar brought by the food that is consumed. When its production is lacking, the blood sugar level increases and affects the organs. There are two types of diabetes: type 1 diabetes, which occurs when the body does not produce insulin, and type 2 diabetes (the most common type of diabetes), which is caused by insufficient insulin production. Over time, too much sugar can cause serious problems that can affect organs such as the eyes, kidneys and nerves. If there are different treatments for diabetes, natural substances obtained from herbs, spices and fruits are fresh, cheap and available everywhere.

Drink a few cups of green tea each day: Green tea is a popular, inexpensive and affordable drink. It contains polyphenol, a powerful antioxidant, and hypoglycemic compounds that help control blood sugar levels and release insulin into the body.

Studies have shown that five to six cups of green tea each day not only protect against cardiovascular disease and cancer, but also improve insulin resistance. Only green tea, however, has these features. Black tea does not count!

Other alternatives: chamomile and basil tea, which are also good for your health . Drink after meals to handle the peak of sugar occurring at this time.

Drink tomato juice or consume at every meal: Studies have shown that 200 grams of raw tomatoes reduce the blood pressure and risk of cardiovascular disease associated with type 2 diabetes.

You can eat raw or cooked. Both are good for your health! Since tomato is a starchy fruit, you can eat as much as you want. You will come to fight cancer and loss of sight!

Eat berries! The berries are rich in vitamin C and antioxidants. They reduce the risk of cardiovascular disease and cancer. Researchers at the University of Illinois have proven that blackberry wine helps reduce and control blood sugar levels.

And they are rich in fiber. Fiber is good for your health! The more you eat, the slower the absorption of sugar by your body. You will find abundant □uantities in apples, oats and carrots.

Use dairy products without fat. If you are already diabetic, this solution will be of little interest. The few studies on the subject showed that people who consumed more dairy products were less likely to have diabetes.

Low fat products are perfect, but those containing no fat are even better. There is a glycemic index classifying all foods containing carbohydrate. The lower the glycemic index, the better the food is for diabetes. Needless to say, non-fat products have a low glycemic

Eat whole citrus fruits. Oranges and grapefruit are an excellent source of fiber, but only if you eat it whole. If you make juice, you just suppress their sugar. With the skin and pulp, they are instead filled with vitamin C.

Collect the onions, garlic and basil. These three foods reduce your bad cholesterol level (low density lipoproteins) and increase that of good cholesterol (high density lipoproteins). This means that the amount of fat present in your blood will decrease and the remaining fat will not clog your arteries . This information sounds like good news.

You can eat these foods as much as you want. The more you add to each meal, the better - as long as your diet is balanced.

Eat fig leaf extracts at breakfast. It must be the first thing to do in the morning. The fig leaves are known for their action against diabetes and their ability to treat diseases such as bronchitis, cirrhosis, high blood pressure, skin problems and ulcers.

Boil a few leaves in a saucepan and drink the resulting herbal tea.

Take 5 to 30 grams of fenugreek with each meal (over 90 grams daily). This spice is hitting the Internet and is the latest trend in healthy products. It turns out that fenugreek reduces cholesterol and blood sugar levels. It also reduces insulin sensitivity. Although fenugreek has these peculiarities, you should consult a doctor before taking any, as it may have side effects such as stomach upset and nausea.

You should not exceed 100 grams of fenugreek a day or take it with other medications. Even if the herbs are really effective, it is wise to consult a professional before consuming.

Turn to ginseng. Some studies have shown that ginseng slows glucose uptake, which is particularly useful when consuming foods high in simple sugar. Ginseng reduces blood sugar levels and helps the body control the amount of glucose absorbed . You will easily find it in the form of tablets at your usual pharmacy.

Just one to three grams of ginseng a day.

Drink half a cup of cinnamon a day. Studies have shown that cinnamon reduces blood sugar levels by mimicking insulin and thus limiting the need for medications that lower glucose levels. It also helps with weight control

The effects of the product are visible in one second. Add more cinnamon to your daily diet for a month and watch how your blood sugar goes down.

Take three capsules of grape seed extract each day. Studies in Japan and the United Kingdom have shown that grape seed extract drastically reduces sugar levels by protecting cells from reactive oxygen species produced under conditions of hyperglycemia.

Make bitter gourd or melon juice. Drink three to six tablespoons (44.4 to 88.7 ml) on an empty stomach every morning. These plants contain p-insulin polypeptide, which is a chemical that lowers blood sugar .

Not very attracted to bitter gourd juice? You can also mix it with curry, however the juice is less diluted and therefore more effective.

How to Change your lifestyle

Change your diet. This is the first thing to do to prevent and treat diabetes. If your blood sugar gets out of control, the only way to stabilize it is to have a healthy and balanced diet. Turn to starch-free vegetables and whole grains that are essential to your diet. Carbohydrates and fats must be consumed in small ⬜uantities.

If you are overweight or obese, it is advisable to lose some weight. Your body, your organs and your arteries do not support excess weight. Even 5 kg of lost can change things!

Consult your doctor regularly. Nothing can replace the advice of a doctor. He can advise you, give you a treatment and suggest an effective diet and exercise program. A professional can help you live well with diabetes.

If there is a history of diabetes in your family, this is a good idea. Diabetes can be hereditary and the sooner you know it, the better you will be.

Ask him for supplements and medications. Even if you do not want to take medicine, there are natural supplements that you can use such as chromium, resveratrol, magnesium.

Drink more water. The thing that comes closest to the miracle on this planet is water. Drink more to lose weight. Drink more to improve the condition of your skin, nails and hair. Drink more to clean your organs and eliminate toxins. Profits will flow as never before. And when it comes to drinking water, it's not about drinking champagne or caloric drinks!

In addition, drinking cold water stimulates 30% of the body within one hour. In addition to daily exercises, go for the H2O!

Know how yoga can help you. There are different yoga exercises perfect for diabetics. They bring back the sugar level to a normal level. Since the exact causes of diabetes are unknown and stress is thought to contribute to its onset as well as its evolution, yoga is practiced to relieve mental and physical stress. It also helps prevent and control this destructive condition.

Adopt Pranayama pose. Sit on your yoga mat with your legs crossed and your back straight. Once in this position, keep your hands straight so that they touch your knees with open palms.

Close your eyes and take deep breaths. Long breaths and exhalation stimulate the pancreas and increase insulin levels in the body.

CHAPTER 4

Diabetic Nutrition and Meal Planning In Action

Diabetic nutrition, diet, and weight control are the foundation of diabetes management. The most objective in dietary and nutritional management of diabetes is control of total caloric intake to maintain a reasonable body weight and stabilize the blood glucose level. Success of this alone is often with reversal of hyperglycemia in type 2 diabetes. However, achieving this goal is not always easy. Because nutritional agreement of diabetes is so complex and a registered dietitian who understands diabetes management has major responsibility for this aspect of therapeutic plan. Nutritional management of diabetic patient includes the following goals stated by American Diabetes association, Evidence-Based Nutrition Principles and Recommendations for the Treatment and Prevention of Diabetes and Related Complications, 2002:

Provide all the essential food constituents like vitamins and Minerals needed for optimal nutrition.

- Meeting Energy needs
- Maintaining reasonable weight

Avoidance of huge daily fluctuations of blood glucose level, with blood glucose level close to normal as is safe and practical to reduce risk or prevent the possibility of complications

Decrease serum lipid levels to reduce the risk of macro-vascular complication

For those diabetic people who require insulin to help control blood glucose levels, maintaining as much consistency as possible in the amount of calories, and carbohydrates ingested at the different meal time is essential. Additionally, precision in the approximate time intervals between meals with the addition of snacks as necessary helps in preventing the hypoglycemic reaction and maintaining the overall glucose control.

For obese with type 2 diabetes, weight loss is the key treatment. Obesity associated with an increase resistance of insulin is also a main factor in developing type 2 diabetes. Some obese who requires insulin or oral anti diabetic agents to control blood glucose levels may be able to reduce or eliminate the need for medication through weight loss. A weight loss as small as 10% of total weight may significantly improve blood glucose. In other instances wherein one is not taking insulin, consistent meal content or timing is not as critical. Rather, decreasing the overall caloric intake assume most importance. However, meals should not be skipped. Pacing food intake throughout the day places more manageable demands on the pancreas.

Long-term adherence to meal plan is one of the most challenging aspects of diabetes management. For the obese, it may be more realistic to restrict calories only moderately. For those who have lost weight, maintaining the weight loss may be difficult. To help diabetic people incorporate new dietary habits into lifestyle, diet education, behavioral therapy, group support and ongoing nutrition counseling are encouraged.

Diabetic Nutrition Meal Plan

Diabetic Meal plan must consider one's own food preferences, lifestyle, usual eating times, ethnic and cultural background. For those who are under intensive insulin therapy, there may be greater flexibility in timing and content of meals by allowing adjustments in insulin dosage for changes in the eating and exercise habits. Advances in insulin management permit greater flexibility schedules than previously possible. This in contrast to the older concept of maintaining a constant dose of insulin and re□uiring the a diabetic person to adjust his schedule to the actions and duration of the insulin.

The first step about meal planning is thorough review of a diet history to identify eating habits and lifestyle. A careful assessment of weight loss, gain or maintenance should also be undertaken. In most circumstances, those with type 2 diabetes re□uires weight reduction.

Diabetic meal Planning [The Making]

In teaching about meal planning, you must coordinate with a registered dietitian and if possible he must use educational tools, materials and approaches so you can fully grasp the idea of your nutritional re□uirements. Your initial education approaches the significance of consistent eating habits, the relationship between the food and insulin and the provision of an individualized meal plan. Then in-depth follow-up sessions which focuses on management skills, such as eating at the restaurants, reading food labels and adjusting the meal plan for exercise, illness and special occasion. An instance like there is an aspect of meal planning such as the food exchange system which may be difficult to learn or understand. You may ask him every meeting for clarification or might as well, leave him a message. Just remember that the food system provides a new way of thinking about the food rather than a new way of eating. Simplification as much as possible grants a good understanding during the teaching session and provides an opportunity to assess doubts and a need for repeat activities and information.

Caloric Requirements

Caloric requirements or your calorie-controlled diets are planned by means of calculating your energy needs (individual energy needs that varies in every person) and your caloric necessity based on your age, gender height and weight. Activity element is factored in to provide actual number of calories re□uired for maintenance.

In the Diabetic Exchange List compiled by American Dietetic Association and American Diabetic association 2008, the appropriate amount of calorie controlled diets are depicted but you must approach a registered dietitian to closely assess you with your current eating habits and achieve realistic and individualized goals. This is so important because practically, developing a meal plan should be based on individual's usual eating habits and lifestyle to effectively control the glucose level as well as the weight loss maintenance. The priority for a young patient with type 1 diabetes, for example, should be a diet with enough calories to maintain normal growth and development. Initially, the target aim may provide a higher calorie to regain lost of weight.

Here is a reliable and simple Food Exchange List For Diabetic Meal Planning I got from Diabetes Teaching Center at University of California, San Francisco via Google.

Please Take note of all these and believe that there's no harm in trying!

Diabetic Nutrition Caloric Distribution

Diabetic nutrition in your diabetic Meal Plan also focuses on the percentage of calories that come from carbohydrates, proteins and fats. In general, carbohydrates have the greatest effect on blood glucose levels because they are more quickly digested and converted than other foods.

Carbohydrates

The American Diabetes Association recommends that for all levels of caloric intake, 50% to 60% of calories should be derived from carbohydrates, 20% to 30% from fats and remaining 10% to 20% from protein. Carbohydrates are consisted of sugar and starch. Most of the carbohydrates that are generally consumed came from starch, fruits and milk. Vegetable has also some carbohydrate. All carbohydrates should be eaten in moderation to prevent postprandial high glucose level. Foods high in carbohydrates such as sucrose are not totally eliminated from the diet but should be taken up in moderation up to 10% total calories only because these foods are typically high in fats and lack in vitamins, minerals and fibers.

Carbohydrate counting method is very important because it makes you conscious about your approximate amount of serving. The more carbohydrates you ingested, the more your blood glucose goes up. It is also a tool use in diabetic management because carbohydrates are the main nutrients in the food that influence the blood glucose level. This technique provides flexibility in food choices, can be less complicated and allows more accurate management with multiple daily insulin injections. When developing a diabetic meal plan using carbohydrate counting, all food sources should be considered. Once digested, 100% of your carbohydrate intake are converted to glucose. Around 50% of protein foods (meat,fish and poultry) are also converted to glucose. The amount of carbohydrates in foods is measured in GRAMS so you have to know which foods contain carbohydrates,learn to estimate the number of grams of carbohydrates in each food you eat and sum up all the grams of carbohydrates from every food you eat in order to get your total intake in a day. Examples of common food that contains carbohydrates; potatoes, legumes (e.g peas), corn, grains, dairy products (e.g milk and yogurt), snack foods and sweets (e.g cakes, cookies, deserts), and

Juices (soft drinks, fruit drinks, energy drinks with sugar).

Lets say, you aim 50% of your total calories must come from carbohydrates. One gram of carbohydrates is about 4 calories. So, divide the number of calories you want to get from carbohydrates by 4 to get the number of grams. Example, you aspire to eat 2000 calories a day and get 50% of calories from carbohydrates.

Computation:

- 0.50 x 2000 calories = 1000 calories
- 1000 / 4 = 250 grams of carbohydrates

Take note that there are people who has lower tolerance of physical activity and there are also those who needs low-calorie diets and therefore, the carbohydrates need in every person really varies. In order to further master your caloric intake and your diet, feel free to contact a professional dietitian.

In terms of estimation on the amount of carbohydrates in every serving, you can refer to Food Exchange List or here are some examples taken from the food exchange list:

These Foods contain 15 grams of each serving:

- Biscuit - 1 (1 1/2 inches across)
- Bun (hot dog or hamburger) - 1/2 bun
- Pancake (1/4 inch thick) - 1 (4 inches across)
- Pita bread - 1/2 pocket (6 inches across)
- Waffle -1 (4 inch square or 4 inches across)
- Cooked barley 1/3 cup
- Cooked Pasta - 1/3 cup
- Cooked Quinoa 1/3 cup
- Cooked white or brown rice - 1/3 cup
- Cassava - 1/3 cup
- Corn 1/2 cup
- Green Peas - 1/2 cup
- Animal Crackers 8 crackers
- Rice cakes, 4 inches across 2

- Dried Apple 4 rings

- blueberries 3/4 cup

- dates 3

- Fruit cocktail 1/2 cup

- Mango juice 1/2 cup or 1/2 small

- papaya 1 cup cubed (8oz)

- Grape Juice - 1/3 cup

Although carbohydrate counting is now commonly used for blood glucose management of type 1 and type 2 diabetes, to some extent it affects the blood glucose to different degrees regardless of e□uivalent serving size. Thus, you have to be consciously noticing the fluctuations of your own blood glucose level and take action against any warning signs.

Diabetic Food Pyramid

The Diabetic Food Pyramid is another tool use to develop meal plan. It is commonly utilize for those with type 2 diabetes who have difficulty in abiding with calorie controlled diet. The food pyramid is consist of six food groups: 1.Breads, grains and other starches; 2. Vegetable (non-starchy vegetables); 3. Fruits; 4. Milk; 5. Meat, meat substitutes and other proteins; and 6. Fats, oils and sweets. The pyramid shape was chosen to emphasize that the foods in the largest area, the base of the pyramid (Starches, fruits and vegetables) are the lowest in calories and fats and highest in fiber and should make up the basis of the diet. For those with diabetes and as well as the general population, 50% to 60% of daily caloric intake must be from these three groups. As you move up the pyramid, foods higher in fats (particularly saturated fats) are illustrated; these foods should account for a smaller percentage of daily caloric intake. The very top of the pyramid comprises of fats, oils and sweets that should be sparingly by the people with diabetes to attain weight and blood glucose control and to reduce the risk of cardiovascular disease.

Fats and Diabetes

The recommendation regarding the fat content for the diabetic diet include both reducing the total percentage of calories from far sources to less than 30% of the total calorie and limiting the amount of saturated fats to 10% of total calories. Additional recommendations include limiting the total intake of dietary cholesterol to less than 30 mg/day. This approach may reduce risk factors such as elevated serum cholesterol levels, which are associated with the development of coronary heart disease, the leading cause of death and disability among people with diabetes. The meal plan may include the use of some non animal sources of protein to help reduce saturated fats and cholesterol intake. In addition, the amount of protein intake may be reduced to those who have early signs of renal disease.

Fiber Has a Lowering Glucose power

The use of fiber in diabetic diets has received an increased attention as the experts study the effects on diabetes of a high carbohydrate, high fiber diet. This type of diet plays a role in lowering the total cholesterol and low-density lipoprotein cholesterol in the blood. Increasing fiber diet may also improve blood glucose and decrease the need for exogenous insulin.

There are two types of dietary fibers: soluble and insoluble. Soluble fibers in foods such as legumes, oats and some fruits plays more of a role in lowering blood glucose and lipid levels than does insoluble fiber. Soluble fiber is thought to be related to the formation of a gel in the gastrointestinal tract. This gel slows stomach emptying and the movement of food in the upper digestive tract. The potential glucose lowering of the fiber may be cause by the slower rate of glucose absorption from the foods that contain soluble fibers. Insoluble fiber is found in whole grain breads and cereals and in some vegetables. This type of fiber plays more roles in increasing stool bulk and preventing constipation.

One risk involving the increase of fiber intake is that it may require adjustment of insulin dosage or oral anti diabetic agents to prevent hypoglycemia. If fiber is added or increase in the meal plan, it should be done gradually and with the actual consultation with a dietitian.

Misleading Labels

Food labeled as "sugarless" or "sugar-free" may still provide calories equal to the equivalent sugar-containing products if they are made with nutritive sweeteners. Hence, for weight loss, these products may not always be useful. Additionally, you must 'not' consider them as "free" to be eaten in unlimited quantity because they may elevate your blood sugar. Foods labeled "dietetic" are not necessarily reduced calorie foods. They may be lower in sodium or have other special dietary uses. They may still contain significant amounts of sugar or fats. Snack foods with labels like "Health Foods" may often contain carbohydrates like honey, brown sugar, and corn syrup. Additionally, these supposedly healthy snacks frequently has saturated vegetable fats, hydrogenated vegetable fats or animal fats which may be contraindicated if you have elevated blood lipids level.

So read the nutritional labels carefully to count the nutrients that your food contains...

Sweeteners

Using sweeteners can be acceptable for the diabetic people especially if it assists their overall dietary adherence. Moderation in the amount of sweetener used is encouraged to avoid potential adverse effect. There are two main types of sweeteners: nutritive and non-nutritive. The nutritive sweeteners contain calories and non-nutritive sweeteners have few or no calories in the amounts normally used.

Nutritive sweeteners include fructose (fruit sugar), sorbitol and xylitol. They are not calorie free; they provide calorie in amounts similar to those in sucrose (table sugar). They cause less elevation in blood sugar levels than sucrose and are often in "sugar-free" foods. Sweeteners containing sorbitol may have a laxative effect. Non-nutritive sweeteners have minimal or no calories. They are used in food products and are also available for table use. They produce minimal or no elevation in glucose level. Saccharin contains no calories. Aspartame (Nutra Sweet) is package with dextrose; it contains 4 calories per packet and losses sweetness with heat. Acesulfame-K (Sunnette) is also package with dextrose; it contains 1 calorie per packet. Sucralose (Splenda) is a newer non-nutritive, high intensity sweetener that is about 600 times sweeter than sugar. The Food and Drug administration has approved it for use in baked goods, non alcoholic beverages, chewing gums, coffee, confections, frosting and frozen dairy product.